Eat Like A Boss

By Jazmin Truesdale

ISBN-13: 978-0-9997284-2-0

Warning:

This book is intended to be a reference guide to a healthier eating lifestyle. If you are suffering from an illness please seek the help of a medical professional.

Table Of Contents

Introduction

The statistics state that over 60% of Americans are overweight and 2 million are obese. Health-care costs are rising and with the current political climate leaving many people questioning the future of their health insurance, the future can seem uncertain for some. While it may seem like there are many things happening that are out of your control, there is one thing that you can control.

Your diet.

The true definition of a diet is not a fad. It is merely the total sum of the food that you consume. Essentially, a diet is any and everything that you are putting in your mouth.

Think about the kind of food you typically eat. Is it lots of fruits and vegetables? Lean meats? If you so, then you have a relatively healthy diet. If you are one of the millions of people who follow the typical American diet, then you have found this book just in time.

This book is not here to judge you or tell you what you are doing wrong. It is merely a guide to help you make the best food choices for you and your body. The body thrives on moderation. Balance. If you give your body what it needs to function at an optimum level then you'll be able to indulge in your favorite guilty pleasures and still maintain all your hard work.

Fad diets are basically eating lifestyles that went viral. They're here today and gone tomorrow. Fad diets were never intended for you to follow long-term. Often times you'll find that if you follow them long-term you'll end up with health problems and vitamin deficiencies.

This book will help you develop a sustainable eating lifestyle so that you obtain all of the nutrients your body needs to achieve your health goals and maintain them. When you are done with this book you will never have to follow a ridiculous fad diet ever again.

Part I

Chapter 1

How To Build Your Plan

Step 1

Make a list of all the things you would like to focus on.

Tips: Be specific. Weight loss is not specific. You should indicate fat loss and/or increase lean muscle.

Sample list:
- Fat Loss
- Anti-inflammation (fluid/swelling)
- Joint health
- Skin health

Step 2

Follow the meal guide as outlined in the book. The Meal Guide is a simple breakdown to help you organize your meals for the day. You can design your meal guide based on your lifestyle, budget, and physical needs. The guide that you design is for your body only because only you would know best what your body needs. After a few weeks the system of eating that you created will be like second nature to you.

Step 3

Read the Basic Food List and start building your plan! For people with special diets (lactose-free, gluten-free, etc.), you will be advised on how to incorporate key nutrients into your plan that are missing from your eating lifestyle. Otherwise, follow the Basic Food List as is.

Step 4

Read through the rest of the book to learn how to eat for your goals. Each chapter/section will teach you about the issue you are trying to improve as well as provide you with an easy-to-follow layout on how to incorporate the necessary foods into your plan. Just plug and eat!

Tip: Chapter 11 contains Meal Tips and Must-haves if you need help organizing your plan or want to know when the best time to eat certain foods is. Preparation of food is entirely up to your discretion (See Chapter 11 for guidance). The plan is designed to help you develop the habit of eating the right foods at the right times for optimal weight management.

Step 5

Don't forget your cheat meals and treats! It can be difficult to bounce back from an entire day or weekend of cheat-eating. For this reason, we recommend 2-3 cheat meals/treats a week. Cheat meals/treats teach you balance so that if you are eating properly throughout the day, your body will be able to handle a cheat meal/treat. Psychologically, you will be able to enjoy the meal without food guilt and it also prevents junk food binge-eating.

Yes! You can have your cake and eat it too...just don't eat the whole cake!

Remember: A slice of apple pie is a treat. The #6 at Popeye's is a meal. If you eat the two together that is two of your three cheat meals/treats for the week.

Chapter 2

Carbs, Proteins, and Fats...OH MY!

The meal guide is designed for you to obtain your carbohydrate, fiber, and protein requirements throughout the day. The fats are based on your discretion and health needs.

Carbohydrates

This is the most important part of your plan and should make up about 60% of your diet. The meal guide is designed so that if followed, you will accomplish this. Most people recognize carbohydrates or "carbs" as breads, whole grains, starches, etc. Carbs also include fruits and vegetables but for the purpose of this book, 'carbs' will be used to refer to pasta, breads, etc. The categories are separated in the meal guide because each meal should contain some sort of fruit and/or vegetable as well as some sort of "filling" or complex carb.

Carbohydrates will fuel your energy, control your hunger throughout the day, and give you that "full" feeling when you eat. For this reason, your largest carb portion should be at breakfast and as the day goes on each meal should contain fewer carbs. Carbohydrates later in the day become optional depending on when you exercise. The meal you eat before exercising should always contain a carbohydrate in order to fuel energy for your workout.

Summary

- **Eat fruits and/or vegetables at every meal.** You can alternate each meal or eat fruits in the morning and vegetables in the afternoon.
- **Eat the majority of complex carbs in the morning and afternoon.** Eat little to no carbs in the evening unless you are exercising)
- **Always eat a carb in the meal prior to your workout to fuel your energy.**

What About Fiber?!?!?

Fiber is naturally a part of the carbohydrate family. If you follow the guide and incorporate fruits and vegetables into every meal and complex carbs during the day you will achieve your fiber requirement.

Two Kinds of Fiber

Soluble: Dissolves in water and forms a gel that slows down digestion. This helps you to feel fuller longer and may aid in the stabilization of blood sugar and insulin in the body. It also helps to lower cholesterol by inhibiting the absorption of cholesterol through food sources.

Soluble Fiber Food Sources

- Oats
- Soy
- Some beans
- Some fruits and vegetables

Insoluble: Does not dissolve in water and allows food to pass through the digestive tract more quickly and therefore preventing constipation.

Insoluble Fiber Food Sources

- Whole grains
- Lentils
- Most beans
- Seeds
- The skins of fruits and vegetables (eat your peels)

Why Is Fiber Important?

- Prevents constipation and contributes to regular bowel movements
- Lowers risk of colon cancer
- Aids in preventing bacterial appendicitis
- Helps in lowering cholesterol which will help reduce the risk or severity of cardiovascular disease
- Can also help with hemorrhoids and bowel disorders

Proteins

This is the most important nutrient that fuels your muscles. Protein sources are also the most crucial part of the diet for people who do not eat meat regularly. The food lists, as well as the supplement guides, are available to you in order to help you determine what protein sources are best for you.

Be sure that you are getting adequate protein for exercise and increasing your metabolism. The protein must be complete with all nine essential amino acids that aid in the digestion of carbohydrates so that you can utilize them for energy. If you chose to not use the recommended protein supplements be sure that the amino acids in the product are clearly labeled so that you know what you are getting.

Protein should be eaten regularly throughout the day and has already been incorporated into the meal guide. However, when taking a protein supplement, for best results take your protein supplement within the first 30 minutes after your workout for faster recovery.

Summary

- Food lists and supplement guides contain recommendations for protein sources
- Be sure that your protein supplements contain the nine essential amino acids. Amino Acids are listed in the Protein section of the book.
- Take protein supplements within the first 30 minutes after your workout for faster recovery
- To determine how many grams of pro-

tein you need: Your body weight in lbs/2.2 (ex. 135lbs/2.2=61.36 or 61 grams of protein a day)

Fats

This is what everyone is trying to burn off. However, fats are needed in the diet because they provide insulation for the body and its organs. This section will be brief because all you need to know is that there are good and bad fats so you should eat more of the good fats...plain and simple.

Good Fats

Unsaturated fats help increase HDL (good cholesterol) and help lower the risk or severity of heart disease. (e.g., Omega 3, 5,6,7,and 9) This would be your fish oils, olive oils, canola oils, etc. You will learn more about fatty acids and how to incorporate them into your diet later in the book.

Bad Fats

Saturated and Trans fats increase LDL (bad cholesterol) and contribute to cardiovascular disease. You can see these on the labels of food products. It's best to keep this fatty acid to a minimum in the diet. For example, try cooking with olive oil instead of butter.

✳✳✳

You should now be aware that your meals should consist of a complex carb, fruit and/or vegetable, and a protein source. The Jazmin Fitness Meal Guide in the next chapter more clearly outlines this. Once you have looked over the meal guide you can then start building your plan through the food lists. There are different food lists for different eating lifestyles (pescetarian, vegetarian, etc.). Find the one that fits your lifestyle and start building.

Part II

Chapter 3

How Your Metabolism Works

Humans are creatures of habit. For that reason, the body functions in the exact same way. If you eat very little throughout the day then your body will respond accordingly with a slow metabolism. If you eat constantly throughout the day then your body will respond with a fast metabolism. That is why it is recommended that humans eat **4-6 meals** throughout the day at **3-4 hour intervals**.

No, this doesn't mean that you should eat McDonald's 6 times a day. However, fueling your body with the nutrients that it needs allows you to boost your metabolism so that you don't have to kill yourself in the gym.

That's right! Your nutrition will be doing the work for you!

The meal guide will be your tool for creating your nutrition plan based off of whatever your fitness goals may be. Each meal has a requirement that needs to be met for an optimal metabolic rate. Carbohydrates, proteins, and fats all play a part in your nutrition and need to be balanced in order to burn fat and lose weight.

There is no need to count calories because fruits and vegetables are naturally low in calories. Nutrition is not all about calories. It's about your body's ability to quickly and efficiently convert food into energy. That can only be done when you are giving your body the nutrients it needs to function properly.

There is a big difference between eating a 1,000-calorie meal full of protein, vegetables and whole grains vs. a 1,000-calorie box of donuts. The first meal has nutritional value while the donuts are nothing but empty calories. Empty calories do nothing for your body. They usually get stored in your body in some unwanted way (e.g., usually as fat or in your arteries).

The main reason why Jazmin Fitness doesn't promote calorie counting is because it doesn't take into consideration the fact that your metabolism can *increase*. When your metabolism increases you'll notice that your normal portions of food are not enough. You'll also find yourself getting hungry more often.

This is a very good thing!

Your hunger is a perfect indicator of what your metabolism is doing. If you find that you're not getting hungry throughout the day, that could be an indicator of a slow metabolism or something more serious like anemia. Hunger is merely your body's way of telling you that it needs fuel. But instead of picking up potato chips, you can try picking up a banana or an apple instead.

Just like you train your muscles with exercise, you can train your metabolism as well. Most fad diets tell you to cut calories. If your body burns 2,000 calories/day and you only eat 1,000 calories, you are going to lose weight. What they don't tell you is that your metabolism will eventually slow down to 1,000 calories/day. So when you go back to eating normally, you will end up gaining all the weight back and more because you now have a slower metabolism. You start dieting again, the cycle repeats itself, and that is what the fitness industry calls yo-yo weight.

This book is going to help you increase your metabolism so that you not only burn fat but you are able to maintain the weight that you've lost.

No more yo-yo weight!

Here is the meal guide that you will be following. Read it carefully so that you can understand how your meals should flow in a single day.

Meal Guide
Meal 1 (Breakfast) Protein Vegetable/Fruit Carbohydrate (Largest Portion)
Meal 2 (Snack) Protein (optional) Vegetable/Fruit Carbohydrate
Meal 3 (Lunch) Protein Vegetable/Fruit Carbohydrate
Meal 4 (Snack) Protein (Optional) Vegetable/Fruit Light Carbohydrate (Optional)
Meal 5 (Dinner) Protein Vegetable/Fruit Little to No Carbohydrate
Meal 6 (Optional) No Carbohydrate

Meal 6?

You're probably wondering what the deal is with Meal 6? Meal 6 is an optional meal that is strictly *No Carb*. It is specifically for people who still feel hungry before going to bed or are trying to gain more lean muscle mass. It can also be for people who need to catch up on whatever nutrients they may have missed during the day.

The meal guide looks like a lot but in a few weeks, this schedule will become like second nature to you. During the first few weeks, you're going to feel full. That's natural. Most people are not eating this often. However, don't worry! As explained before, you are training your body to be able to process food more quickly an efficiently. It's going to take a week or two for your body to adjust. In approximately 3-4 weeks you're going to notice your stomach growling every 3-4 hours. That means your metabolism is increasing!

Note

Carbohydrates are what your body uses as an energy source to fuel digestion and the metabolic process; therefore, carbs should not be eaten before bed because your body is going into a state of rest.

Chapter 4

Basic Food List

This is your basic food list to get you started on building your plan. For vegetarians, vegans, lactose-free, etc. you can find your accommodated food lists in the next chapters.

Remember: This book is designed to teach you HOW to eat not tell you WHAT to eat.

Building a meal is simple. Just pick any food from the following categories and plug them into your meal template. From there, you can do whatever suits your tastes. Create your favorite stew and add key foods you never thought to add or modify a recipe by substituting ingredients. You can even try creating your own recipes. If you are dining out you can look for dishes that contain the foods you need and have it modified to your liking.

Basic Food List

Protein

Chicken
Beef
Lamb
Turkey
Goat
Legumes (beans, nuts, seeds, lentils)
Quinoa (S) (H)
Eggs
Dairy
Pork
Seafood

Vegetables

Carrots
Potatoes (any kind)(H)
Beets
Turnips (H)
Onion (any color)
Asparagus
Leafy Greens (the darker the better)
Peppers (any color)
Zucchini
Kale (S)
Broccoli

Carbohydrate

Quinoa (S) (H)
Oats (S)
Whole grains (especially breads and pastas)
Rice
Potatoes (S)(H)
Turnips (H)
Squash (any kind) (H)
Bulgur

Fruits

Pomegranates (S)
Banana (S)
Apples
Oranges (juice does not count)
Cherries
Berries (cranberries, strawberries, etc.)
Tomatoes (yes, they are a fruit)
Mango
Peach
Pear
Avocado (S)

Meal Example:

- Protein: Salmon
- Carbohydrate: Sweet Potato
- Vegetable/fruit: Dark Green Salad with red, yellow, and green peppers, red onion, olive

oil and balsamic vinegar

Turkey is an excellent source of protein but lacks the amino acid variety of chicken. If you eat mostly turkey be sure that you are also including some sort of complete protein supplement in your plan.

Hybrid foods: As mentioned before, carbohydrate is a very broad category and has been simplified for the purpose of this book. If you eat a hybrid food such as a potato, which is a starchy root vegetable, be sure to include some other non-hybrid vegetable or fruit source. Hybrid foods are great bread/pasta replacements if you want to cut back on gluten.

Superfoods: These are amazing foods that are jam-packed with key vitamins, minerals, and/or proteins. You will learn all about superfoods later in the book.

Chapter 5

Lactose/Casein-Free

Surprisingly, this is not an uncommon accommodation. There are many people who are intolerant or at least sensitive to lactose, especially in adulthood. If you are having any inflammatory issues such as asthma, eczema, digestion, hemorrhoids, etc. try decreasing or eliminating cow products in your diet.

Cow products are a bit more difficult to digest and can also take longer to go through your system. This affects your body's ability to absorb nutrients and can also affect your immune system. The effects do not just come from by-products such as milk, cheese, and yogurt but also beef. This is especially true for people who have difficulty digesting the protein casein.

The biggest issue with the lactose-free diet is

finding a suitable calcium replacement. Fortunately, there are many alternatives and they are listed below. In addition to the basic food list, the lactose-free food list is designed to emphasize the right foods into your plan to assure that you are getting your daily **calcium**.

(S)Superfood; (H)Hybrid Food

Protein
*Same as basic food list; *if you are casein-free you should avoid beef
Salmon
Almonds
Sesame Seeds
Legumes (Soybeans, white beans)
Carbohydrates
*Same as basic food list
Fortified Cereals
Oats-Fortified (S)
Vegetables
*Same as basic food list
Kale (S)
Dark Leafy Greens
Seaweed
Fruit
*Same as basic food list
Oranges

Dairy Alternatives
Goat Dairy
Sheep Dairy
Substitute milks (Almond, soy, etc.)
Coconut (milks and yogurts)

Goat Dairy

Goat is the best animal dairy substitute and is consumed by a large portion of the world population. It is the closest thing to human breast milk which automatically tells you that it will be much easier to digest. If you are allergic to cow's milk then there is a 50% chance that goat will be the best alternative for you. If you can digest goat's milk than your issue is not with lactose per se but the protein casein that is found in all cow products.

Benefits of Goat Dairy

- Easier to digest
- Contains MCTs (medium chain triglycerides) which help speed up metabolism and lower cholesterol
- Naturally contains less fat than milk
- Provides more calcium and protein than

cow's milk
  • Contains significantly less lactose than cow's milk
  • Usually raised without hormones or antibiotics
  Goat is best suited for people who are lactose sensitive or allergic to casein.

Summary

  • Play with your diet to see if your issues improve when you eliminate or decrease intake of cow products
  • If you are intolerant or sensitive avoid dairy products AND beef
  • If eliminating cow dairy you must replace it with something else to obtain your body's calcium needs

Note

As we all know it can be impossible to be completely lactose/casein free, especially when eating outside of the home. Listed below are some recommended digestive enzymes that can help ease symptoms caused by lactose/casein sensitivities.

Digestive Enzymes

- Enzymedica GlutenEase
- Enzymedica Lacto
- Enzymedica Digest Spectrum

Chapter 6

Gluten-Free

Gluten is now the thing that everyone is talking about when it comes to weight management. The good thing is that because of the buzz, companies are now making more gluten-free alternatives than ever. Typically, a gluten-free diet would be for people who have celiac disease or have difficulty processing the protein gluten; however, many are finding that going gluten-free or "gluten-low" also has its benefits.

Benefits of A Gluten-Free or "Gluten-Low" Diet

• Gluten-free foods tend to be less processed

and contain few if no fillers (but not always)

• Body is better able to absorb nutrients from foods (if you have a gluten sensitivity)

• May improve symptoms of other inflammatory health issues (e.g., eczema, bloating, gas, leaky gut etc.)

Going gluten-free is not a guaranteed weight loss strategy. Remember, you are still eating carbohydrates. However, it may improve digestive issues and inflammation.

Fortunately, meats, fruits, and vegetables are gluten-free in their natural state. For this reason, it is important that you check the labels of processed or packaged foods for hidden gluten or make sure that the product has the certified gluten-free stamp. Below is a short yes and no list you can use as a guide.

'Yes' Ingredients

Amaranth
Arrowroot
Buckwheat
Millet
Flax
Soy
Tapioca
Chia Seeds
Xanthan Gum

'No' Ingredients

Imitation Meats/Seafood
Beer/Malt beverages or condiments
Matzo
Sauces/Dressings (some use gluten as a thickening agent)
Some additives and preservatives
Barely
Rye
Wheat

The biggest issue for gluten-free/low dieters will be eating as clean as possible and finding a good carbohydrate source. Remember to always proceed with caution when eating packaged foods and you can never go wrong with preparing meals at home. Below is a list of carbohydrate food sources; otherwise follow the basic food list.

Carbohydrate

Gluten-free Flours (rice, soy, corn, potato, bean)
Gluten-free breads
Corn and Cornmeal
Potatoes (any kind) (H)
Quinoa (S)
Rice

Summary

- Beware of hidden gluten in packaged foods
- When cutting gluten from the diet be sure to incorporate good carbohydrate replacements (rice, yams/potatoes, vegetable pasta are examples of great complex carbohydrates)
- Try eating as 'clean' as possible (e.g., make your own dressings/marinades)

Note

As we all know, it can be difficult to follow a gluten-free diet when eating outside of the home. Try a digestive enzyme to see if that eases your digestive discomfort. ***Enzymedica GlutenEase*** is an excellent product if you're gluten sensitive.

Chapter 7

Pescetarian

Pescetarian diets can be difficult because not all seafood is created equal. Not every fish is designed to be eaten daily and some seafood should be eaten with caution (e.g., mercury levels, high cholesterol, etc.). The biggest issue with the pescetarian diet is making sure that you have a consistent daily protein source. However, there are many benefits to a pescetarian diet.

Benefits of A Pescetarian Diet

• Excellent omega-3 sources (excellent for decreasing inflammation and lowering cholesterol)

    • Fish tend to be leaner in fat content especially saturated fat (great for fat loss)

    • Fish are excellent protein sources

    • Rich in Iodine (excellent for thyroid health)

Typically pescetarians are viewed as vegetarians who eat fish. For this reason, listed below is a guideline for how to eat fish. You can read the next chapter about the Vegetarian/Vegan lifestyle for alternative protein suggestions. For the carbohydrate, fruit, and vegetable categories follow the basic food list.

Protein

High Mercury (eat with caution)
Swordfish
Shark
King Mackerel
Tuna
Low Mercury (2-4x/week)
Salmon (Wild-Caught)
Flounder
Catfish
Trout
Cod
Scallops

High Cholesterol (1x/week)
Shrimp
Shellfish (e.g., crab, lobster, mussels, etc.)

Tuna is a funny fish. The fresher it is the better. Eating canned light tuna tends to have less mercury. If you are unsure, wild-caught salmon is always an excellent alternative.

Note

• Women who are pregnant or trying to get pregnant can typically eat up to two servings of fish per week. Ask your doctor for more guidance.

• See the next chapter for alternative protein sources for when you are not eating fish.

• Proceed with caution when eating fish with high mercury levels.

Chapter 8

Vegetarian/Vegan

There is no further explanation for this particular eating lifestyle, simply put...you don't eat meat and if you're vegan then you don't eat meat by-products. For obvious reasons, the biggest issue that a vegetarian/vegan will have is finding a protein source. Luckily for you, there are plenty of vegetarian/vegan protein and amino acid supplements to assist with this.

It is highly recommended that you do both a food source and protein supplement to ensure that you are getting all the protein (amino acids) that you need in a day. For example, seeds, nuts, beans, and quinoa are excellent protein sources. Later in this book, you will also receive guidance on the best protein supplements.

Another issue that vegans and vegetarians run

into is anemia. Key nutrients for blood building include zinc, iron, and B12. These are best
absorbed through meat sources but there are
ways around this. You will learn all about best
food and supplement sources for this in the blood
building section of the book.

Below is a protein food list. All other categories are the same as the basic food list.

Protein
Quinoa (S)
Whole Grains
Legumes (Beans, Lentils, etc.)
Soy
Tempeh
Nuts and Seeds
Animal Dairy (Vegetarians)

Chapter 9

No Red

This section is specifically for people who don't eat red meat. While you are able to get excellent sources of protein one of the main things that you will be lacking are key blood-building components such as B-complex and iron as well as zinc. You will learn all about best food and supplement sources for blood-building later in the book.

In the meantime, follow the basic food list as normal but here some great zinc food sources for you.

Zinc Food Sources

Protein
Nuts and Seeds (Sesame, pumpkin, sunflower)
Seafood (Crab, Scallops)
Beans
Vegetables
Spinach
Kale
Leafy Greens
Carbohydrates
Oats
Wheat Germ
Whole Grains
Brown rice (be cautious of arsenic levels in brown rice)

Note

Be careful when taking zinc supplements. There is such a thing as too much. The upper limit for zinc is 50mg; taking more than that can cause nausea and digestive issues. Supplements should not be more than 50 mg and even then you should only take half of the dosage.

Supplements should 'supplement' food not replace it. If you are taking high doses of zinc you may also want to take copper. Over time zinc supplements can inhibit the absorption of iron, especially in high doses. Taking copper can help correct this.

Chapter 10

Superfoods To The Rescue

These are the foods that are jam-packed with awesome nutrients to help fuel a meal. If you find yourself missing key nutrients throughout your day then these are the foods for you. Even if your eating habits are excellent, it never hurts to have a few superfoods in your meal arsenal. Below, are examples of superfoods and why they are so... super.

Apricots

This fruit is like nature's gummy bear. Dried apricots are sweet and delicious as well as nu-

tritious. They are loaded with fiber, vitamin A
(eyes), vitamin C (immune health), vitamin E
(skin and hair), as well as potassium (excellent for
lowering blood pressure.)

Avocados

There is so much to say about this amazing
fruit (yes it is a fruit). It is loaded with fiber,
various B-vitamins (blood building, hair growth),
Vitamin K (blood building), and potassium (blood
pressure). It is also an excellent source of ome-
ga-3 (anti-inflammation) as well as good cholesterol.

Bananas

This fruit is a great carbohydrate booster between meals. It is an excellent source of potassium (blood pressure), fiber, Vitamin C, manganese
(overall health), electrolyte source (hydration),
and prebiotic (promotes healthy stomach bacteria).

Beans

Beans are an excellent gluten-free vegetarian

source of protein, fiber, iron (blood building), potassium (blood pressure), manganese, B Vitamins, and zinc (body repair/healing). They also contain properties that are excellent for increasing metabolism and burning fat.

Berries

These fruits are rich in antioxidants which help rid the body of free radicals and therefore, aiding in the prevention of various cancers, premature aging, and common illnesses (flu). Their richness in color also makes them excellent for anti-inflammation. However, the most important berry for women is the cranberry because they help cleanse the kidneys and may aid in the prevention of UTIs (urinary tract infections).

Broccoli

This is an excellent detox vegetable due to its antioxidant properties that help to cleanse the liver and other parts of the body for optimal health. It is known for its cancer-fighting and anti-inflammatory properties. It is also an excellent source of various B-vitamins, manganese, fiber, Vitamin C, A, and K, potassium, and many other micronutrients.

Citrus Fruits

These fruits are known for their antioxidant properties especially around flu season. They are also good for promoting collagen production in the body which is great for preventing premature aging, improving joint health, skin/hair health, preventing hemorrhoids, and improving the overall molecular structure and functions of the body. Citrus fruits are excellent sources of folate (B-vitamin/blood building), potassium, fiber, and other excellent micronutrients.

Garlic

Not only does garlic add flavor to food but it also serves as a natural antibiotic. Cooking vegetables with fresh garlic and olive oil can be a great way to boost your immune system.

Molasses (Blackstrap)

No, this isn't a food but it has so much going on that it must be mentioned. It is an excellent source of iron, calcium, magnesium, potassium, copper, manganese, and other micronutrients. It is also an excellent condiment for breads/pastries or sugar substitute when baking.

Oats

This is a heart-healthy carbohydrate that is excellent for lowering bad cholesterol. There are gluten-free varieties...just be careful of the labeling. Oats are jammed packed with vitamins and minerals making them an excellent super-food.

Pomegranates

Pomegranates are a powerful super fruit that can aid in the prevention of many cancers. Its antioxidant properties help to remove free radicals from the body and help to fight premature aging.

Potatoes

Sweet or not, potatoes are an excellent hybrid food serving as a good vegetable source as well as a filling carb due to its starchiness. It is an excellent **resistant carb** that promotes an increase in metabolism to help you lose weight. It is naturally gluten-free and is an excellent source of fiber, potassium, hyaluronic acid (joint, skin/hair health), vitamin C, and manganese.

Quinoa

This gluten-free pseudo-grain is considered a hybrid food serving as an excellent protein and carbohydrate source. With its anti-inflammatory properties, it also contains magnesium, folate, phosphorus, and manganese as well as other micronutrients.

Salmon

This fish has it all. It is an excellent protein source loaded with omega-3, phosphorus, selenium, vitamin D, and various B-vitamins (particularly B-12). Salmon is perfect if you need an energy boost and you are looking for something healthy and lean.

Sea Buckthorn

This fruit is incredibly bitter but contains extremely powerful antioxidant properties that help rid the body of free radicals that contribute to illness and premature aging. You'll learn more about this fruit in the Omegas section of this book.

Nuts & Seeds

Nuts and seeds are not only good protein sources but also loaded with vitamins and minerals, particularly sunflower seeds and pumpkin seeds.

• Sunflower Seeds – vitamin E, manganese, copper, magnesium, selenium, phosphorus, B-vitamins

• Pumpkin Seeds – manganese, iron, zinc, copper, phosphorus, magnesium

Squashes

This hybrid vegetable is gluten-free as well as low in fat, carbs and cholesterol. It is rich in magnesium, vitamin A, potassium, fiber, vitamin C, and lutein (eye health). So try making spaghetti using spaghetti squash instead of noodles or make a butternut squash soup to fuel your meal.

Tomatoes

This fruit is super easy to find. Tomatoes are excellent for many reasons. They are rich in vitamin C, A, and K, fiber, various B-vitamins, manganese, potassium, magnesium, and copper. Although tomatoes are abundant in the American diet it never hurts to know what makes them so awesome!

Chapter 11

Meal Tips and Must Haves

A lot of information has been thrown at you about how to build your plan. This page is devoted to simplifying the process even further by giving you some tips and tricks as well as some advice on things that MUST be included in your plan.

Program Design

The program was designed for you to easily plug in key foods and obtain your daily requirements of protein, complex carbohydrates, and vegetables/fruits for weight management. This book is here to teach you how to eat so that you can achieve your goals and maintain your hard work. Over time, you will develop a habit of knowing which foods are best for you and your needs and, essentially, not even have to look at your plan. This will take time but you will get there.

Meal Breakdown

Each meal is broken down into three categories that need to be fulfilled to be considered a meal. Simply go to the basic food list and there will be a list of foods already categorized for you. All foods listed under protein can be plugged into the protein section of your meal, all carbohydrates in the carbohydrate section, and so on and so forth.

Building a meal is that easy.

Preparation of the meal is entirely up to you and your tastes. The important thing that this book is trying to instill is that you develop the **habit** of eating healthy and learn how to make your nutrition complete.

Meal Tips

• Eat your largest portion of carbohydrates in the morning and afternoon while avoiding 'heavy' carbs in the evening (helps to control hunger and energy).

• Evenly distribute fruits and vegetables throughout the day. You can alternate them with each meal or eat all your fruits in the morning and veggies in the evening.

• Plan a meal 1-2 hours before your workout that contains a good energizing complex carbohydrate (fruit, vegetable, complex carb)

• If taking a protein supplement, take it within 30 minutes after your workout

• Eat something GREEN at some point in your day. *Every day.* Leafy greens are super important and should be incorporated into your plan, daily.

• Get creative with your plan. There are plenty of options so that you are not eating the same thing every day.

• Soups, stews, and casseroles are amazing because they allow you to include many vegetables and meats together for an amazing dish. They can also help you save money if you make enough to last multiple days. Try making a vegetable/meat stew with all your important foods.

• Smoothies are excellent for obtaining fruit and vegetable servings. Make sure you are using real fruits and vegetables and not just juices when making your smoothies.

• Limit your sugar intake. Try using honey, agave, or even molasses as sugar substitutes.

Must-Haves

Must-haves are things that must be included in your plan for optimal weight management. The plans have been designed for you to easily incorporate must-haves into your diet without skipping a beat. Just plug and eat!

• Omegas-3,6,9 – definitely a must. Keeping a balance of this is most important to control inflammation.
• Complete proteins or protein supplements containing essential amino acids.
• Vitamin D – very important for absorption of calcium, energy, hormone regulation, and cancer prevention.
• B-vitamins – along with an iron source and amino acids/protein will be your best friends for energy and increasing your metabolism
• Probiotics – helps to keep your bowels regular and good bacteria in your system for a high functioning immune system. This can be difficult for people on a lactose-free diet but not impossible.

This may seem like a lot but truly it is only a matter of developing a plan that works for you. There are many vitamin sources that overlap with others and don't forget about Superfoods. You will notice that the meal template is all encompassing to allow you to easily fit all of these things into your day.

Chapter 12

Meal Preparation Tips

Benefits of Preparing Your Own Meals

• You have the freedom to prepare meals exactly to your tastes

• Save money

• No hidden ingredients (you know exactly what you are putting in your food–excellent for people with food allergies)

• You can modify recipes to fit your health and fitness goals

Tips for Preparing Meals

- **Don't be afraid of substitutes!** In fact, get creative! Just because a recipe requires butter doesn't mean the recipe is no good. Try using olive oil instead.

- **Discover the world of flavor.** Getting creative with seasonings makes it so that you are not dependent on salt. Actually, a pinch of salt can go a long way with the right seasonings.

- **GLUTEN-FREE:** Don't be afraid of stews because of the flour content! Try using Sweet Rice Flour to make the roux needed to thicken the stew.

- **Don't get caught in the fast food trap!** Yes, it's convenient but so is having food already made in your refrigerator. Try to cook enough food to last you multiple days. This will help you save money and keep you from relying on fast food.

Part III

Chapter 13

Supplement Guide

We see these everywhere from Walmart, to GNC, to the Vitamin Shoppe. Everyone is telling you about the supplements you should take but no one actually tells you when to take them, what they work best with, and what they don't. This section is designed to help you know what supplements you need to take to achieve your fitness and health goals. Each supplement is broken down into categories of what you are trying to achieve (e.g., increase muscle mass, blood building for anemia, etc.)

Each Section Contains:

- Explanation of the supplement and the

health issue
     • The best supplements for that issue and how to take them
     • The foods to eat in conjunction with those supplements
     • Foods are broken into categories just like before so that you can easily fit them into your plan. Start eating with a purpose and tackle whatever health issues you have.

Supplement Basics

Read the next section on Multivitamins to see if they are right for you.

Supplements are designed to supplement nutrients that are missing from your diet not replace food altogether. That is why each section contains a food list. If it is possible to incorporate a food source into your plan it will lessen the need for a supplement.

Not all supplements are created equal. Raw food source supplements are always highly recommended because your body recognizes them better than artificial supplements.

Example: Let's take an artificial iron capsule containing 18mg of iron. The capsule contains 100% of the recommended daily dose of iron but your body only recognizes 20% of it. Basically, you are throwing 80% of your money down the toilet.

Also, there is absolutely NO NEED to be taking 1000% of any particular vitamin unless you are deficient in it or completely lacking it in your diet because you cannot eat the food source. Vitamins have upper limits. This means that you can only ingest but so much of a vitamin before you start to have problems. It is very possible to get too much of a good thing. Remember your body needs to be in balance so try not to overdo it.

The purpose of a supplement is to mimic whatever the food source it is you are lacking.

Example: Taking a B-complex with an iron-rich meal would be the equivalent of eating a steak for a vegetarian. Try to take vitamins that work well with certain foods whenever you can.

A list of recommended daily allowances is always available on the Jazmin Fitness website. It lists the recommended daily amount of important vitamins and nutrients as suggested by the National Institutes of Health. Keep in mind that daily amounts vary by age.

Multivitamins

Multivitamins are made to provide you with all the essential vitamins and nutrients you need in a day. The average person usually will see a multivitamin and say, "Score! I get everything I need in one pill!" This has been the mentality for many years especially now that the quality of food is going down. The reality is that people are not designed to obtain nutrients in that way for any extended period of time. While multivitamins are convenient they can also be ineffective at times. This is because there are many nutrients that inhibit the absorption of others.

One prime example is calcium and iron. These two nutrients are probably the most important nutrients you will need because your bones hold your skeletal structure together and iron replenishes your blood to keep your body functioning. However, ironically both nutrients inhibit the absorption of each other when taken in high doses. For example, taking your main iron supplement for the day with milk would be counterproductive. As most people know, calcium is better absorbed with vitamin D. However, many people don't know that iron is better absorbed with vitamin C . The same thing applies to food. Eating foods with certain other foods can increase the absorption of key nutrients. So next time you take an iron pill, try taking it with orange juice.

When to Use A Multivitamin

• When traveling (e.g., vacation, for work) and you are unable to maintain your normal diet.
• When buying a multivitamin is more cost effective for you (sometimes buying individual vitamins can be expensive)
• If you are a child. Children can be fickle about what they are willing to eat which can affect their nutrient intake.
• If the product contain only 50-100% of the most essential vitamins. (Recommended)

If the product only contains 50-100% of the essential vitamins, you will still need to EAT the rest of your nutrients. This is highly recommended because you do not become reliant on the multivitamin. Some people see multivitamins as a substitute for eating healthy which should never be the case. Eating is the only way to increase your metabolism and lose fat.

The best time to take a multivitamin is in the morning with breakfast. This will fuel your energy for the day and allow you to prepare your meals to essentially supplement whatever you are not absorbing from the multivitamin. The superfoods section of this book provides you with many amazing multi-vitamin food sources.

Suggested Multivitamins

Vega One: all-In-OneNutritional Shake
• All Plant-based sources
• Great absorption
• Contains vitamins, protein, omega-3, probiotics, and fiber
• Gluten, Soy, and Dairy Free
• Comes in great flavors!
• Provides 50% of essential vitamins
Garden Of Life: Raw Meal
• Comes from raw plant sources
• *Best absorption rate!!*
• 2 scoops replaces a meal; 1 scoop can be used as a snack or add to a meal
• Provides 50%-100% of essential vitamins
• Contains vitamins, probiotics, fiber, protein, and digestive enzymes
• Gluten, Soy, and Dairy Free; Vegan
• **CON:** Although an extremely effective supplement it is not the best tasting so you will have to dress it up to your liking. Trying blending with a 100% fruit juice and/or frozen fruit

Vitamin Code: Women
- Gluten and Dairy Free
- Raw vegetable sources
- Contains vitamins, probiotics, and digestive enzymes
- 50-100% of hard to obtain vitamins and low in calcium and iron making it effective for absorption with calcium/iron-rich meals
- Available for women over 50
- Vegetarian
- **CON:** you must take 4 capsules to obtain all nutrients

Rainbow Light: Women's Multivitamin
- Organic vegetarian sources
- Recommended: only taking 2 capsules instead of 4; other nutrients can be eaten
- low in calcium and iron making it effective for absorption with calcium/iron-rich meals
- **CON**: Recommended for people who eat meat/animal dairy

These supplements have the best absorption rates and are free of most allergens. Of course, if you don't have any food sensitivities you have many more product options.

Protein

Protein supplements and protein sources are going to be the key to your fat loss or weight management. Protein is essential to the body's functions because its compounds (amino acids) are the building blocks for the body's tissue structure. It is for this reason we stress how important it is that you find protein supplements that are complete proteins.

Complete proteins are considered to have all the essential amino acids. Amino Acids are basically how the body utilizes protein. How it works is that you ingest protein through a food source, the body breaks the protein down into an amino acid which is then utilized for metabolic functions in the body (e.g., breakdown and convert carbs into energy, muscle recovery, building lean muscle mass, etc.). Generally, you will know if a product contains all essential amino acids because the company will brag about it on the label.

Nine Essential Amino Acids

- Isoleucine
- Leucine
- Lysine

- Methionine
- Phenylalanine
- Threonine
- Tryptophan
- Valine
- Histidine

Of course, the more amino acids the better. However, make sure that your protein supplement at least contains the nine essentials.

What To Avoid In Protein Supplements

- Fillers (heavy sugars and other unnecessary ingredients)
- Labels that don't specify all 9 essential amino acids — if the product doesn't name all nine then it doesn't have all nine.
- Hidden allergens (e.g., lactose-free people should avoid whey protein): Soy, dairy, nuts, and gluten are often used in protein supplements so be sure to carefully read the labels

Most people who eat meat will not have an issue with obtaining all the amino acids they need in a day. Vegetarians/vegans will need a supplement because plant proteins tend to lack one if not many essential amino acids. Fortunately, there are plenty of plant-based products that utilize various vegetable and fruit sources to create supplements containing all of the amino acids that you need.

Recommended Protein Supplements

Plant Fusion
• Dairy, soy, and gluten-free
• 21 g of protein per serving
• Provides all essential AAs and more
• Enzymes to assist in digestion
• Comes in different flavors
Garden of Life: Raw Protein
• Gluten-free and Dairy-free
• 17 g of protein per serving
• Great source of Vitamin E, D, K, and A
• Enzymes to assist in digestion
• Probiotics
Country Life: Max-Amino Caps
• Great if you don't like powders
• Hypo-allergenic* (Gluten and Dairy-free)
• Vegetarian-based
• Excellent absorption

Note

Be careful with amino acid supplements in pill form. Many times they will use casein as a pre-digestive enzyme which dairy-free consumers should avoid.

For people who are trying to gain weight or increase mass, try increasing your protein intake.

Make sure you are balancing your protein intake throughout the day. Try not to exceed 20-25 grams of protein per meal. Anything more than this can be really hard on your kidneys and cause damage over time. Your meal guide has already accounted for this. If you need 60g/day, eat 20g of protein at breakfast, lunch, and dinner.

Probiotics

These essentially are good bacteria that assist in immune and digestive health. The world is filled with good and bad bacteria and it's the good bacteria that prevent us from getting sick. The good thing is now that we know about probiotics food companies are starting to incorporate them into more products.

Benefits

- Help control inflammation in the intestines (gas and constipation)
- Aids in calming acid reflux
- Good bacteria provides an excellent defense against common bacteria that make us sick
- Maintain vaginal health (acidophilus)
- Aids in body's ability to absorb nutrients
- Regulate the body after taking antibiotics

There are many good bacteria but acidophilus is essential for women. This particular bacteria helps to keep the vagina healthy. If you notice odor or itchiness, especially after a menstrual cycle, then try taking some acidophilus. Unfortunately, not all probiotics contain this particular culture so it is important that you are reading the labels of your products.

Probiotic Food Sources

- Dairy (yogurt, kefir, milk)
- Non-dairy Yogurts (fortified)
- Sauerkraut
- Kombucha Tea
- Miso soup

Note

Many probiotic products come from milk cultures and other hidden allergens. Make sure that you are reading labels carefully.

Recommended Products

Garden of Life: RAW Probiotics • Excellent probiotic designed specifically for women • Available for women over 50 • Must be kept refrigerated • NOT milk-free but does contain enzymes to help break down casein and lactose (use at your own discretion)
CountryLife: Power-dophilus • Dairy-free probiotic • Contains acidophilus for women and other excellent probiotics • Gluten-free • Must be kept refrigerated
Bluebonnet: Acidophilus Plus FOS • Dairy-free probiotic • Contains acidophilus and other excellent probiotics • Comes in tablet and powder form

Prebiotic Food Sources

- Legumes (beans, nuts, seeds, lentils)
- Oats
- Bananas
- Asparagus
- Artichokes
- Honey
- Red Wine

Prebiotics help probiotics thrive in your system. Many of these foods, you'll notice, have already been listed as sources for other things. It's amazing how nature works like that.

Chapter 14

Omega Fatty Acids

Omega-3 (Fish Oil)

This is the fatty acid that everyone is talking about. Its blood thinning properties make it so that it is excellent for people at risk for cardio-vascular disease. Typically, it comes from oily fish but it can be obtained from other sources for people who don't eat fish. Listed below are some of its benefits for why it is a must-have.

Benefits

- Excellent for anti-inflammation (counter-acts Omega-6) this is great for people with in-flammatory issues like arthritis, eczema, digestive inflammation etc.
- Skin health and hydration
- Improves cardiovascular health
- Improves brain health (helps with mental disorders and improves focus)
- Lowers the risk of certain cancers (particularly breast and colon)
- Reproductive health

This fatty acid is broken down into three different kinds: ALA, EPA, and DHA. Fish oils contain EPA and DHA which is how the body uses omega-3. ALA comes from typically non-fish sources and is later converted into EPA and DHA by the body. However, remember too much omega-3 can be just as bad as too little. The recommended amount of omega-3 intake should not exceed 3g or 3000mg. Too much omega-3 can lead to hemorrhaging.

Follow the basic food guide as usual and here are a few food sources to increase the omega-3 in your diet.

Omega-3 Food Sources

Protein
Seafood (Salmon is an excellent source)
Chia Seeds (S)
Flax Seeds
Hemp Seeds
Walnuts
Eggs (fortified)
Vegetables
Brussels Sprouts
Hummus
Fruit
Avocado (S)

Although there are many omega-3 supplements out there, studies have shown that the most beneficial way to obtain omega-3 is through a food source.

Omega-5 (Pomegranate oil)

You are probably thinking Omega-What?!? Exactly, this is a silent omega that most people have never heard of. Its antioxidant and anti-inflammatory properties are something to sing about and should definitely be incorporated into your plan at least 2x/week.

Benefits

• Extremely powerful antioxidant (excellent in preventing premature aging of the skin) ridding the body of free radicals that affect cardiovascular and skin health
• Aids in the prevention of many cancers (particularly breast cancer)
• Powerful anti-inflammatory properties

Omega- 5 Food Sources

Protein
Wild-Caught Salmon
Grass-fed Dairy (Whole Milk)
Macadamia Nuts
Fruit
Pomegranates (best source)
Oils
Palm
Coconut

*Try adding pomegranates to your favorite

smoothie or muffin recipe for an omega-5 boost!

Omega-6 (The Inflammatory Fat)

This is THE most abundant omega in the American Diet. This particular fatty acid is very much needed for the body's immune response to bruises and injuries but too much of it can just be plain...damaging. Unfortunately, this is a key ingredient in the American diet so basically it is everywhere from packaged/processed foods to the bread that you buy, fast food, and even meat. However, don't freak out! Your body needs omega-6 to properly heal from injuries and assist in the body's immune responses. The important thing is to make sure that you are balancing the omega 3 and 6 in your body. If you find that you are eating a lot of omega-6 (noticeable inflammation and swelling) then you need to also find a good omega-3 source.

We're not going to go into the benefits of Omega-6 but just give you a list of sources. Make sure that you are not over-eating them but instead you are balancing them with omega-3 sources.

These foods are rich in omega-6 and have excellent benefits when used in moderation.

Omega-6 Food Sources

Protein
Nuts and Seeds
Poultry (especially chicken)
Oils
Safflower
Sunflower
Corn
Sesame
Peanut
Soybean (vegetable oil)
Canola
Grape seed
Coconut (S)

When eating nuts and seeds try to eat no more than a handful a day, especially walnuts which have a ratio of 5:1 of omega 6 : 3.

Coconut oil is an excellent superfood just make sure you are using it in moderation.

Omega-7 (Sea Buckthorn)

You've probably heard about this amazing omega from Dr. Oz. Omega-7 does so many things for the body it's amazing no one had heard of it before.

Benefits

- Collagen production
- Anti-inflammation
- Skin health (retaining moisture, rejuvenation, protect against premature aging, sun damage)
- Repairing and moisturizing membranes of the body (including skin)
- Excellent aid for fat loss
- Improves cardiovascular health by decreasing bad cholesterol and improving elasticity of arteries
- Omega 3,6,7 and 9 is naturally found in the sea buckthorn fruit

Omega-7 Food Sources

- Macadamia Nuts
- Sea Buckthorn Fruit

Sea Buckthorn can be found in juice form or oil form. Sibu products or New Chapter are the most recommended.

Omega 9 (Olive Oil)

This particular omega is a non-essential fatty acid because the body is able to produce it in small amounts. However, the body is only able to produce it if you are obtaining a proper balance of Omega-3 and 6. It is for this reason that adding omega-9 sources will help contribute to your omega-3,6,9 balance for optimal cardiovascular health as well as inflammation.

Benefits

- Excellent antioxidant properties
- Anti-inflammatory properties
- Contributes to skin health
- Aids in improving or maintaining cardiovascular health

Omega-9 Food Sources

- Nuts and Seeds
- Avocado (S)
- Olives/Olive Oil (best source)

Omega-9 is in many sources that also contain omega-6 (nuts and seeds). For the purpose of this book, only the most abundant omega-9 sources are listed.

Note

Omega-3,5,6, and 9 have no supplement recommendations because they are very easy to
obtain through diet. Simply adding two tbsp. of
flaxseed or 1 tbsp. of chia seed to your favorite
yogurt will give you an excellent omega 3,6,9 balance. This will save you money in the long run
instead of buying expensive and sometimes ineffective fish oils when you could have easily just
made fish at home.

Part IV

Chapter 15

Anemia/Blood-Build-ing/Fat- Loss

Blood-building is probably the most important thing for a woman and ironically the most over-looked in the female diet. On a monthly basis, a woman loses blood because of her menstrual cycle but how many women are replacing that blood-loss through nutrition?

One big misconception is that iron is going to cure your anemia. Yes, you need iron to build blood but this nutrient does not work alone. Iron works best not only with vitamin C but also B-complex. B-complex (basically a group of B-vitamins) is easy to obtain from diets consisting of red meat but may be difficult for people with special diets such as vegetarians/vegan and no red.

What many people don't know is that blood building is also essential for your metabolism and immune system. When trying to lose fat, B-complex is needed for energy production and improving metabolic functions. Many people notice that when they take a B-complex they find themselves getting hungry more often which is an excellent sign of a high metabolism.

Signs You May Be Iron or B-vitamin Deficient

- Low energy
- Decrease in appetite/or consistent lack of appetite
- Constipation
- Sensitive to cold/constant feeling of being cold
- Do you get sick often? (It's as if you catch every cold and every flu)
- Bruising easily

Anemia can be very tricky because there are so many components to blood-building. Most people assume anemia means iron-deficient when in reality, you could be deficient in B-12. Work with your doctor to determine what your deficiency is.

Blood-Building Food Sources

C (Vitamin C), B (B-complex), I (Iron)

Protein	C	B	I
Salmon and Shellfish		✓	
Squash and Pumpkin Seeds		✓	✓
Nuts		✓	✓
Red Meat (Lamb, beef, etc.)		✓	✓
Poultry (dark meat)		✓	✓
Beans and Lentils		✓	✓
Vegetable			
Dark Leafy Greens	✓	✓	✓
Colored Peppers	✓		
Brussels Sprouts	✓	✓	✓
Mushrooms		✓	✓
Carbohydrates			
Wheat		✓	
Wheat Germ		✓	
Oats - fortified (S)		✓	✓
Quinoa (S)		✓	✓

Fruit	C	B	I
Avocado (S)		✓	
Oranges	✓	✓	
Strawberries	✓	✓	
Guava	✓		
Kiwi	✓		
Grapefruit	✓		
Tomatoes	✓		
Cantaloupe	✓		

Salmon is very rich in B-12.

Tomatoes contain a phytonutrient called lycopene which is considered to be a natural cancer fighter.

B-complex is a large group of vitamins; however, they work best when together. This is why if you are deficient in one B-vitamin you are most likely deficient in others as well. With the exception of B-12, which comes mostly from meat products, most other b-vitamins can come from plant/fruit food sources.

Who May Need B-complex

- Vegans/Vegetarians
- No red eaters

- Anemic
- During/After a menstrual cycle

It is not unusual to take iron and/or b-complex for a couple of days after menstruation in order to recover from blood loss. If you are particularly anemic, taking iron during menstruation has proven to ease cramps and decrease flow.

Recommended Iron and B-complex Supplements

Country Life: Easy Iron
     Hypoallergenic
     Vegetarian Capsules
     25mg of Iron
     Good for taking during/after menstruation or if you are anemic

Country Life Coenzyme B-Complex
     Hypoallergenic
     Vegetarian Capsules
     Contains Soy
     Provides all B vitamins (1 capsule for maintenance, 2 capsules to replenish)

Vitamin Code RAW B-Complex
Vegan Gluten and Dairy-free Provides all B vitamins (1 capsule for maintenance, 2 capsules to replenish)
Vitamin Code Healthy Blood
Vegan Gluten and Dairy free Excellent for during/post menstruation Excellent for anemia Does not contain all B-vitamins 1 capsule for maintenance, 2 capsules to replenish

Note

Taking B-complex with a meal is an excellent way to increase nutrient absorption because B-vitamins help your body break down food and convert it to energy. Make sure you are also drinking lots of water. B-vitamins are water soluble and can cause dehydration if you're not drinking enough water throughout the day.

You'll also notice an increase in appetite. B-vitamins are metabolism boosters. Don't be alarmed! It's a good thing. Your metabolism is increasing. Follow your food guide and eat accordingly.

As mentioned before, avoid taking iron with

calcium and zinc supplements as they can possibly inhibit absorption. Try taking a calcium supplement at breakfast and an iron supplement at lunch or dinner. This will give your body time to process the supplements and maximize absorption. This also applies to multivitamins. If the multivitamin you're taking contains iron, avoid taking it with calcium.

B-12 is also best absorbed when calcium is present. This doesn't mean you have to take B-complex with a calcium supplement. However, if you are eating something rich in calcium like an orange, spinach, or cheese it wouldn't hurt to take a B-complex with it.

B-12 is also best absorbed from a meat source. So if you're eating a steak, try adding a salad with spinach or steamed kale for the calcium component.

Chapter 16

Bone-Building

Bone building is important to women at all stages in their lives. Why? So that you can either prevent osteoporosis as you get older or lessen the severity of the condition now that you are older. As most people know, calcium is essential to bone building and the body uses vitamin D to absorb it. It is for this reason orange juice and milk tend to be fortified with vitamin D.

What many people don't know is that the body uses the calcium stored in bones for many metabolic functions so it's important that you are replacing it with supplements and/or food sources. Other nutrients that are excellent for bone-building besides Vitamin D are magnesium and vitamin K.

Vitamin D

Obtaining this particular vitamin can be tricky because many people spend the majority of their time inside or wear sunblock when outdoors. 20 minutes of sunlight a day without sunblock to absorb vitamin D is typically recommended. Unfortunately, melanin or skin pigment can affect how much vitamin D you absorb because it naturally protects you from the sun. For this reason, people with darker complexions are recommended to take some sort of vitamin D supplement. This is something you should ask about during your next check-up; most times vitamin D levels are not checked unless requested or you have a history of deficiency.

Benefits of Vitamin D

- Regulation of hormones
- Lowers risks of developing cancer
- Increase hair growth
- Increase energy levels
- Improve immune health
- Improve bone development (you need vitamin D to absorb calcium)
- Anti-inflammatory properties

Vitamin D is fat soluble so it is best taken with

a fat source such as meat/meat products, high fatty acid foods (omega 3,6, and/or 9).

Magnesium

This is a mineral that assists other key nutrients that are absorbed by the body. Deficiency in this can lead to osteoporosis, migraines, high blood pressure, muscle spasms, cardiovascular disease (magnesium is key to maintaining heart rhythm), among other things. Fortunately, this is easy to obtain through diet.

Vitamin K

This vitamin is key for blood coagulation (clotting) and preventing the fracturing of bones. If you think that you are bleeding excessively during menstruation increasing the vitamin K in your diet may help with this. Vitamin K is SUPER easy to obtain through diet by simply eating green vegetables. For this reason, eating something green every day is included in the list of must-haves.

*Animal Dairy is the best source of calcium as most people know. You can find additional calcium food sources in the lactose/casein-free food list mentioned earlier in this book. Here are the food sources for other bone-building nutrients.

Bone-Building Food Sources

D (Vitamin-D), M (Magnesium), K (Vitamin-K)

Protein	D	M	K
Salmon and Tuna	✓		
Nuts		✓	
Beans and Lentils		✓	
Vegetable			
Dark Leafy Greens		✓	✓
Fortified Juices	✓		
Carbohydrates			
Fortified Cereals	✓	✓	
Whole Grains	✓	✓	
Bran		✓	
Fruit			
Avocado (S)		✓	
Bananas		✓	
Fortified Juices	✓		
Other			
Molasses (S)		✓	

*Limit or avoid caffeine, foods high in sugar,

and alcohol. Especially when eating calcium-rich meals.

Recommended Supplements for Bone-Building

Rainbow Light: Sunny Gummies

Allergen safe
    Excellent absorption
    Excellent taste
    1000 IUs of Vitamin D3
    Also comes in raspberry flavor with 2500 mg of D3

Garden of Life: RAW D3

Vegetarian, Gluten-free, Dairy-free
    Best absorption
    5,000 IUs of Vitamin D3

Vitamin Code Grow Bone System

System that provides all that is needed to grow bone
    Gluten and Dairy-free
    Contains Soy (fermented)
    Raw food sources
    Probiotics and digestive enzymes
    Contains Silica (excellent for hair and skin)

> **Rainbow Light: Food-based Calcium**
>   Gluten and Dairy-free
>   Excellent absorption
>   500 mg of Calcium per serving
>   Provides vitamin D and magnesium
>   Provides horsetail and silica (excellent for skin and hair)

You've probably seen soy mentioned in a few of the supplements. For those of you who do not have soy sensitivities, you will read all about soy later in the book.

Note

The body only absorbs about 500mg of calcium at a time so taking 1000mg of a calcium supplement may be counterproductive. Try to cut the pill in half or split intake between food and supplements.

Chapter 17

Skin and Hair

Your skin, the largest organ of your entire body, also needs the most care. We use everything for it from lotions, oils, and butters to keep it smooth. But how many are actually eating to keep their skin healthy? One thing is for certain your skin is a reflection of what is going on internally. Your skin shows how hydrated you are, whether or not you are ill, allergic reactions, and even stress. Basically, your skin is like a best friend who can't keep a secret.

The reason for skin issues can vary depending on the person; therefore, it is important that you are aware of your body so that you notice changes before they become a serious problem. The key to skin health is maintaining overall health.

Ways to Improve Skin Health

- Getting rest
- Exercise (sweating helps to eliminate toxins from the body, exercise also helps tone the muscles so that your skin stays firm)
- Eating balanced meals
- Finding positive ways to eliminate and handle stress
- Building your immune system to prevent illnesses
- Drinking plenty of water
- Limiting excessive sun exposure (Too much sun can definitely be bad for you)

These are all things that you've heard before but taking care of yourself as a whole is the key to skin health and preventing premature aging. Your hair is also an extension of your skin so healthy skin also means healthy hair.

Vitamins for Skin & Hair

- **Vitamin C** (antioxidant and helps with collagen production)
- **Vitamin E** (antioxidant and helps with skin moisture, blood circulation, and healing/repair)

- **Omega-7** (Moisturizes the skin and boosts collagen production, anti-inflammatory properties)
- **Omega-3** (Moisturizes the skin, anti-inflammatory properties)
- **Omega-5** (Powerful antioxidant that assists in prevention of premature aging)
- **Iron** (Deficiencies can cause brittle hair, baldness, and dry skin)
- **Iodine** (Helps with metabolism and detoxification, necessary for optimal thyroid health)
- **Hyaluronic Acid** (moisturizes the joints, skin, eye health)
- **Zinc** (Healing and repair, great for skin and scalp conditions, anti-inflammatory properties)
- **B-complex** (Blood building and circulation for skin moisture and hair growth)
- **Vitamin A** (maintain skin moisture, healing/repair, anti-inflammatory properties)
- **Protein** (Specifically amino acids; Collagen is a protein made up of amino acids. Making sure you get all your essential amino acids allows your body to be able to produce it.)
- **Silica** (excellent for skin and hair–found in bamboo, horsetail, fruits and vegetables)

Yes! It's a lot but don't panic because you've tackled most of this list already. Many of these vitamins and nutrients have already been discussed in other sections so you are already heading in the right direction. Also, don't forget many of these food sources overlap each other so don't stress over making sure you get everything.

Example: Sweet Potato = Carbohydrate/ Vegetable hybrid food, Vitamin A, and Hyaluronic acid

Tip: Soups, stews, and casseroles are amazing because they allow you to include many vegetables and meats together for an amazing dish. They can also help you save money if you make enough to last multiple days. Try making a vegetable/meat stew with all your important foods.

You probably noticed a new word. Collagen. Collagen is a protein that contributes to the structure and elasticity of your skin, hair, and nails. If you want to maintain a healthy youthful glow, decrease the appearance of wrinkles, and prevent premature aging then collagen is what you need. While there are collagen products you can take, it is possible for you to eat in a way that your body is able to produce it on its own. Getting your body to produce collagen naturally is the *true* secret to maintaining a youthful look.

Healthy Skin & Hair Food Sources

A (Vitamin-A), I (Iodine), HA (Hyaluronic Acid), E (Vitamin-E)

Protein	*A*	*I*	*HA*	*E*
Sunflower Seeds				✓
Seafood		✓		
Almonds				✓
Eggs		✓		
Dairy		✓		
Soy (fermented)		✓		
Vegetable				
Dark Leafy Greens	✓			✓
Seaweed		✓		
Carbohydrates				
Sweet Potato/Yam	✓		✓	
Butternut Squash	✓		✓	
Root Vegetables			✓	
Fruit				
Avocado (S)				✓
Papaya	✓			
Apricots (S)	✓			✓
Cantaloupe	✓			

Other	A	I	HA	E
Animal Bones (Broth)			✓	

Fruits/Vegetables grown in iodine-rich soil can provide you with iodine in your diet. Unfortunately, this isn't consistent nor is there an efficient way for you to check. It would be wise to not to use fruits and veggies as your main iodine source.

Root vegetables are very starchy veggies like potatoes, turnips, beets, parsnips, carrots, cassava, ginger, onions, etc. They're rich in antioxidants and their starchiness makes them an excellent carbohydrate source.

Animal parts or bones have excellent HA content. Usually, you can find this in broths. Try making a homemade meat broth or when using meat to season foods don't remove the bones.

***

While it is recommended that you eat for your skin and hair health, sometimes you may need a little boost. Below is are supplements highly recommended for you.

Recommended Supplements

Garden of Life: Collagen Builder
Vegan
Gluten-Free
Great Absorption
A variety of plant extracts for maximum effect
Life-Flo Liquid Iodine Plus
2-3 drops provides all iodine needed for the day
No taste
Easy absorption
No allergens

****Note****

Many collagen products are created from meat sources. Make sure that you are reading labels carefully.

Chapter 18

Anti-Inflammation

Inflammation is part of the body's immune response. When you hurt your knee it inflames in order to heal the injury; however, too much or chronic inflammation can contribute to serious health issues. It is also something that many people are not thinking about in their diet. Any type of disease that contains –itis at the end of the word is caused by the inflammation of something.

- **Dermatitis** – inflammation of the skin (eczema)
- **Hepatitis-** inflammation of the liver
- **Colitis** – inflammation of the colon/large intestine
- **Arthritis-** inflammation of the joints

Omega-6, as mentioned previously, is what causes inflammation in the body and while omega-6 is needed in the diet for immune response, too much of it can lead to serious health issues. Unfortunately, omega-6 is hidden in just about anything you can imagine and for that reason, it is important that you are balancing the omega-3 and 6 in your body through diet. The omegas section provides a list of food to help you maintain that balance.

Tips to Limit Inflammation

• *Limit the amount of packaged or processed foods in your diet.* They usually contain a lot of sodium, filler ingredients, omega-6 oils and other things that cause inflammation.

• **Make sure you're getting enough Omega-3**. Omega-3 is important to anti-inflammation.

• *If you can make something at, home by all means, do it!* Sweet potato fries are always better when they are homemade. Making things at home allows you to control the ingredients in your foods and save money.

• *Limit the salt in your diet.* Salt causes inflammation by forcing the body to retain water or "water weight". A good way to balance this is by increasing the potassium in your diet.

   • *Eat more colorful fruits and vegetables.* Not only are they pretty but they also contain excellent anti-inflammatory properties.

   • *When cooking try using olive oil instead of vegetable oil.* Vegetable oil is usually made from soybean oil which can do more harm than good when it comes to inflammation and overall health. If you have to use vegetable oil try to at least cut back on how often you use it.

Anti-inflammatory Food Sources

Protein
Salmon/Tuna (Omega-3)
Chia Seed/Flax Seed
Vegetable
Carrots
Colored Peppers
Red Onion
Beets
Garlic
Dark Leafy Greens
Carbohydrate
Sweet Potato

Yam (any color)
Colorful Squashes (Butternut, Spaghetti)
Whole Grains
Fruit
Banana
Apples
Tomatoes (S)
Avocado (S)
Pomegranate (S)
Sea Buckthorn (S)
Pineapple
Orange
Berries (Strawberry, Blueberry, etc.)

Garlic is also a natural antibiotic which is excellent for fighting colds and common illnesses. Try incorporating fresh garlic into simple dishes for a boost in your immune system.

Note

You'll notice that many of these foods overlap with other foods that are good for other issues. For this reason, fruits and vegetables are such an essential part of every meal. Change it up! Mix it up! There are plenty of choices out there.

Chapter 19

Blood Pressure

High blood pressure is an issue that is plaguing many Americans, particularly the African-American and Hispanic communities. This section will help to educate you on what contributes to high blood pressure and what you can do about it.

You'd be amazed to know that 1/3 of people who have hypertension have no clue that they even have it. This is terribly dangerous because untreated hypertension can lead to other diseases/complications such as kidney disease, atherosclerosis, heart disease, eye diseases, preeclampsia (pregnancy), and diabetes among other things.

Symptoms of High Blood Pressure

- Headaches
- Fatigue
- Confusion
- Vision problems
- Difficulty breathing
- Arrhythmia (irregular heartbeat)
- Hematuria (blood in urine)
- Pounding sensation in the chest, neck, and/or ears

If you suspect that you may have high blood pressure then definitely see your doctor to be sure. This book should not be used a substitute for seeing a medical professional.

Blood Pressures Ranges

	Systolic/Diastolic
Low	90/60
Normal	120/80
Pre-hypertension	120-139/80-89
High: Stage 1	140-159/90-99
High: Stage 2	≥160/100

Ways That May Help Control or Prevent Hypertension

- **Trim your waistline.** Studies have shown that women with excessive adipose tissue (fat tissue) around their waistline tend to be at a higher risk for hypertension.
- **Exercise.** Regular exercise can help to lower high blood pressure. The Jazmin Fitness website provides various exercise plans for you and your fitness goals!
- **Eat a diet rich in fruits, vegetables, and whole grains.** 3 out of 4 Americans do not eat enough fruits and vegetables. Just imagine the amount of money you would save in health-care costs simply by eating properly.
- **Balance your cholesterol.** Cholesterol and hypertension go hand in hand. Limit high-fat cheeses and saturated fats in your diet.
- **Lower the sodium in your diet.** African-Americans have been shown to have a high sensitivity to salt. Try eating less processed foods and using less salt in home-cooked meals. By increasing the Potassium in your diet you can counteract the effects of salt on your blood pressure.
- **Try not to drink excessively.** Although red wine has been shown to have positive effects on blood pressure, too much alcohol can have the

opposite effect.

Excellent Potassium Food Sources

Protein
Legumes (Beans, Lentils)
Vegetable
Swiss Chard
Spinach
Mushrooms
Root Vegetables
Kale (S)
Green Vegetables
Bell Peppers
Carbohydrate
Potatoes
Yams
Squashes
Fruit
Bananas
Papaya
Tomatoes
Avocado
Oranges

| Grapes |
| Apricots |

Note

There are no supplement recommendations for this section. Lowering blood pressure and cholesterol require lifestyle changes.

Chapter 20

Achy Joints

Joint health is something everyone needs to be concerned about, especially as they grow older. There are many things that contribute to the function of a joint and for that reason, you must make sure that you are taking care of your body in more ways than one.

Common Joint Problems

• Dryness- creaky joints similar to a door that needs its hinges oiled.
• Pain – particularly when performing actions of strength such as climbing stairs or lifting heavy objects
• Inflammation – arthritis, swollen joints

As you can see, some of these things are issues we have discussed in previous sections. That is why joint health is all-encompassing and it is important that you are taking care of your body as a whole.

What Contributes to Healthy Joints?

• **Hyaluronic acid and silica**, as mentioned in the Skin Health section, not only works to lubricate the skin but also the joints which prevent that creaky feeling.

• **Collagen** production for the skin also helps to maintain the structure of the bones, ligaments, and tendons that make up a joint.

• **Bone-Building** is important as well not only for preventing osteoporosis but to help support the bone structure in a joint which can help eliminate pain and inflammation.

• **Exercise** is important to strengthen the muscles that help stabilize the joints. If you are not active and you find that you have weak knees you may also have weak leg muscles. Your thigh muscles (quadriceps) help to stabilize the knee and prevent injury. Movement also helps to lubricate the joints (that's why trainers want you to warm up before exercising). All of the exercise plans on the Jazmin Fitness website incorporate stability exercises for strong joints.

• **Stretching**, which most people overlook, helps to prevent muscular imbalances that contribute to chronic pain in joints such as the lower back and knees.

• **Inflammation** is the source of arthritis pain. For this reason, it is important to maintain the balance of Omega 3 and 6 in your body. The inflammation causes pressure and stresses the joint which contributes to the pain.

• **Glucosamine and Chondroitin** are great for maintaining healthy cartilage. Typically chondroitin comes from shellfish and bovine/cow sources so it's important that you are paying attention to labels if you have allergies or are vegan/vegetarian.

Recommended Supplements

Deva Vegan Vitamins Glucosamine
Vegan sourced
Contains Glucosamine but not Chondroitin
Still provides excellent joint support and lubrication

Doctor's Best Glucosamine Chondroitin MSM with OptiMSM

Contains Glucosamine, Chondroitin, MSM, and Collagen sources

Chondroitin comes from bovine (cow)

Non-vegetarian

Country Life Glucosamine Chondroitin

Non-vegetarian

Excellent source for Glucosamine and Chondroitin

Shellfish based

Chapter 21

Cholesterol

Cholesterol...sigh...this is a silent killer that develops over time and can be very difficult to manage. Unless you're reading this book which will definitely help you with that. There is no need to go into detail about cholesterol except to say that there are two different kinds: Good (HDL) and bad (LDL) and you obviously know which one to increase and which one to decrease.

What makes bad cholesterol so BAD is that over time it builds in the arteries causing blockage that can lead to strokes, arteriosclerosis (hardening of the arteries), among other fatal heart illnesses. Lowering bad cholesterol is a lifestyle change. Eating more fruits and vegetables will help but unless you are decreasing your intake of bad cholesterol through better eating habits then your cholesterol numbers are not going to change.

Key Habits to Lower Bad Cholesterol

• Decrease or eliminate your intake of fried/oily/fast foods

• Eggs are high in cholesterol. Be careful to balance eggs in your diet. Don't eat eggs for breakfast and then fried chicken for dinner. Try eating just the egg whites which are high in protein without the cholesterol.

• Limit intake of saturated fats (whole milk, butter, cheese)

• Decrease intake of high cholesterol seafood. This was explained in the pescetarian food list.

• Limit red meat and pork (no more than once a week)

• Be careful with snacking. Many packaged/processed foods are high in cholesterol. Try making homemade snacks or buying snacks with very few ingredients.

• Make sure you are getting 25-30 grams of fiber a day. The meal plan has accounted for this. If you are eating fruits and vegetables throughout the day, you will easily achieve this.

Food Sources for Managing Cholesterol

- Any fruit
- Any vegetable
- Whole grains
- Fermented soy
- Foods rich in Omega Fatty Acids (especially 3,5,7, and 9)

****Note*****

There are no supplement recommendations for cholesterol because lowering cholesterol is a lifestyle change.

Chapter 22

Thyroid Health

It is not a secret that women are more suscep-
tible to thyroid issues than men. Yet, for some
reason women, who enter the doctor's office with
the suspicion of there being something wrong
with their thyroid are often sent home being told
that they are fine. Well in this section we are
going to tell you some excellent ways to eat for
thyroid health. Granted, if you suspect there may
be something wrong please see a doctor.

The Thyroid Is Responsible For:

- Energy

- Metabolism
- Regulation of hormones
- Sleep
- Calcium balance
- Body Temperature

Key Nutrients for Thyroid Health

- Iodine – Essential nutrient for the thyroid; helps the thyroid perform all its necessary functions
- Selenium – Another essential nutrient for the thyroid to help in all necessary functions
- Zinc – Necessary for production of thyroid hormones, when zinc is low usually your thyroid hormones are low as well
- Iron – Low iron can decrease thyroid function and therefore slow metabolism
- Copper – Assist in body's ability to produce thyroid hormones
- B-complex – Help the body produce T4 (a thyroid hormone)
- Vitamin A, Vitamin C, Vitamin E – Antioxidant vitamins that you may remember from the skin health section. Antioxidants eliminate stress from the body by removing free radicals that contribute to illness, disease, and premature aging.

Healthy Thyroid Food Sources

S (Selenium), C (Copper)

Protein	S	C
Seafood	✓	
Sunflower Seeds (S)	✓	✓
Brazil Nuts	✓	
Cashews		✓
Organ Meats (liver, kidneys)	✓	
Tempeh		✓
Legumes (beans and Lentils		✓
Carbohydrate		
Wheat	✓	
Rice	✓	
Oats	✓	

Goitrogens

These are some foods that may contribute to a decrease in thyroid function when over-consumed in RAW form. For the average healthy individual as long as they are getting a variety of fruits and vegetables this is something you do not have to worry about.

- Root vegetables

- Broccoli, cauliflower, cabbage
- Collards, mustard, kale, bok choy
- Strawberries, peaches

Balance is key! Too much of a good thing can sometimes be bad. Most of us eat goitrogens in cooked form which lessen their potency; however, if you suffer from an iodine/selenium deficiency or hypothyroidism you may just want to be careful of your intake.

Read the next chapter to learn how soy can affect your thyroid as well.

Chapter 23

Soy

It's a lovely vegetable with excellent health benefits but too much of it can have negative side-effects. The truth is that soy is good for you when processed a certain way or eaten in moderate quantities. Surely no manufacturing company is going to tell you that because it would hurt the sales of their products since soy is in just about... EVERYTHING. From packaged foods to lotions and hair care products soy is almost inescapable.

Almost.

What most people don't know is that the majority of the soybeans used to make products are genetically modified and sprayed with pesticides; unless the food label states otherwise. Also, soy naturally contains anti-nutrients that when over-eaten can cause adverse health problems such as vitamin D and B12 deficiencies, exposure to MSG and aluminum, blood clotting, and thyroid issues in women like hypothyroidism and thyroid cancer, among other things.

Soy also is a phytoestrogen. There are many phytoestrogen foods but soy (and maybe flaxseed) should be the highest on your priority list. Basically, it's imitation estrogen that blocks "normal" estrogen and when over-consumed it can increase the risk of developing endocrine problems, infertility, and cancer. Now imagine all the products that you consume daily that contain soy. That means the bread you eat, processed meats, packaged foods, vegetable oil, soy milk, tofu, lotions, shampoos/conditioners (yes, your body absorbs everything you put on it)...you name it.

Most people are consuming these products multiple times a day giving your body a phytoestrogen overload! Plus 75% of Americans don't eat enough fruits and vegetables that provide the body with fiber and detox nutrients that can help rid the body of all this excessive estrogen.

So what soy is good soy?

Fermented Soy

The process of fermented soy from organic soybeans is natural and helps neutralize the anti-nutrients so that your body can benefit from all the great things about soy. This includes preventing cardiovascular disease, cancer, and osteoporosis.

Fermented Soy Sources

- Natto
- Miso
- Tempeh
- Soy lecithin (organic)

Note

Cutting back on soy and flaxseed may be most beneficial to women who suffer from or have the potential of developing fibroids. It is understood that estrogen feeds the development and growth of fibroids. Women naturally produce estrogen. Cutting back on phytoestrogens, may help with fibroid pain, decrease the size of fibroids, or even prevent fibroids.

Chapter 24

Stomach Acid, Acid Reflux, Food Absorption

Stomach Acid plays a major role in your body when it comes to digestion. Stomach acid allows your body to break down the food that you eat so that you can absorb nutrients through the walls of your intestines. Many people are aware of what happens when their body produces too much stomach acid, but do you know what happens when your body doesn't produce enough?

When your body produces too much stomach acid, you develop symptoms of acid reflux. This is what happens when stomach acid doesn't stay in your stomach like it should. The acid will come up through your esophagus and many people can even taste it in the back of their mouth. You'll feel a burning sensation in your throat and chest area and in extreme cases it can feel like you're having a heart attack. Often acid reflux is easily controlled through antacids...but what happens when your symptoms don't go away?

If you find yourself suffering from frequent acid reflux and antacids don't seem to be helping, you might be suffering from too little stomach acid. The symptoms of too little/too much stomach acid are exactly the same so most people are not even aware of the problem. Fortunately, there are small home-based tests you can do to determine your issue.

Stomach Acid Test

Mix 6oz of water with ¼ teaspoon of baking soda on an empty stomach first thing in the morning. After 5 minutes if you haven't burped, you may be suffering from too little stomach acid

Symptoms of Low Stomach Acid

- Heartburn
- Indigestion, diarrhea, constipation

- Bloating and flatulence immediately after meals
- Rectal itching
- Undigested food in stools
- Acne

You're probably wondering why any of this matters. The truth is that if you're not producing enough stomach acid then you're probably not absorbing the nutrients from the foods that you're eating. Imagine that you are ingesting iron-rich foods and supplements in order to counteract your iron-deficiency anemia. If you have low stomach acid then your body will not be able to properly absorb the iron. In many cases, low stomach acid could be the reason why you have anemia in the first place.

That's right! Your body's inability to absorb nutrients due to low stomach acid can contribute to nutrient deficiencies and malnutrition. Fortunately, there are many ways to help your body produce more stomach acid.

Ways to Produce More Acid

- ***Apple Cider Vinegar*** - ACV helps to balance the pH of your stomach. Taking a shot of ACV before meals can help with digestion.
- ***Lemon water*** - Lemons and other diges-

tive bitters are great for helping to stimulate the production of stomach acid. Sugar is in EVERY-THING and is probably why an estimated 40% of Americans experience symptoms of low stomach acid. Lemon water naturally cleanses and detoxifies the body, gives you a boost of vitamin C, and is an inexpensive way to make alkaline water. Drinking lemon water before and during meals can aid in digestion.

• *Digestive Enzymes* - we've already discussed enzymes earlier in the book but they can also help with low stomach acid symptoms.

• **HCL and Pepsin** - This is the quickest solution but should also be taken with care. HCL/pepsin is very strong and can cause problems if not taken properly. Many HCL/pepsin supplements are made from pork and other animals so definitely read the labels if you are vegan/vegetarian. Fortunately, vegetables don't require much stomach acid to digest so any of the natural remedies mentioned above will do just fine. Everyone's stomach acid levels are different so working with a medical practitioner is the safest way to determine your correct dosage.

• *Following the food guides -*   There are many vitamins and minerals that contribute to the body's ability to produce healthy levels of stomach acid (e.g., iodine, zinc, B vitamins). This creates an interesting catch-22: Low stomach acid is preventing you from absorbing the nutrients you need to produce more stomach acid. Unfortunately, the only way to fix this is with time.

Time. Time is the only thing that is going to fix this issue. If you're taking an HCL supplement you'll notice that you need less and less until you don't need it anymore. Over time, your stomach acids will normalize and you'll be able to produce stomach acid naturally. Your energy levels will increase, bowels will pass more smoothly, and you'll even notice significant fitness gains.

Chapter 25

Detoxing

Detoxing. People talk about this constantly when referring to weight loss. "Drink this and the fat will just melt away." "This detox program will destroy fat in 30 days!" Blah, blah, blah. It's all a load of crap. They're selling you the Brooklyn Bridge. It's a gimmick.

Marketers are counting on the fact that most people don't know anything about how their body works. They also know that most people are not going to do the research necessary to catch them in their lie. It's all an elaborate scheme to take advantage of unsuspecting consumers and make money.

A detox's only function is to cleanse you. Nothing else. It's the equivalent of scrubbing the ring around your tub after taking a bath. Cleansing is not the same as losing weight. If you lose weight during a detox it is most likely water weight or gunk clogging up your intestines. Not Fat.

But don't get discouraged!

Detoxing is a good thing. It's an excellent way to give your body a fresh start. Your body goes through a lot every day. It's constantly working and sometimes we do things to it that makes it have to work even harder. Just like an engine in a car every now and then your body needs a tune-up.

Everyone knows that eating junk food is bad. Everyone also knows that eating poorly can make you gain weight. Did you know that it can also clog the lining of your intestines?

Eating fruits and vegetable not only provides you with vitamins and nutrients but they also provide you with fiber to eliminate waste from your body. What makes junk food so bad is that it has a lot of empty calories and useless ingre-dients that the body can't (or shouldn't) process. When you eat junk food it is broken down in the stomach and absorbed through the intestines. Whatever your body can't process will cling to the walls of your intestines. Normally, this in-testinal waste will find its way into your toilet if you get enough fiber (e.g., fruits, veggies, and whole grains). However, 75% of Americans don't eat enough fruits and vegetables and they surely don't get enough fiber.

Now just imagine all of the gunk that can cling to an intestinal wall after months or years of eating a poor diet with very little fiber.

Yikes!

That is why detoxing is important. You can accumulate so much gunk in your intestines that you develop a pot-belly in your golden years (yes, Grandpa). That gunk also prevents you from absorbing nutrients and getting the most out of the healthy foods that you're eating.

Reasons to Detox

- Fasting gives your organs a rest
- Helps the liver to clean out toxins
- Helps the body eliminate waste through the skin, intestines, and kidneys
- Gets rid of parasitic organisms living in your intestines

Yes, you read that correctly. Parasitic organisms!

Almost everyone has them; especially, if you eat meat or have ever eaten meat. They hook onto your intestines and grow by eating everything that you eat. Again, eating enough fruits, vegetables, and whole grains can help them find their way to the toilet but a detox can help kill off the stubborn ones.

There are many products on the market that help with intestinal parasites but Jazmin Fitness recommends Dr. Natura. The products are healthy, natural, and they even have a detox system for the kidneys and liver. Bam! You're welcome.

Warning! A Detox is only intended to last for a short time. Anywhere from one day to thirty days depending on the intensity of the program. Detoxing every 3-6 months depending on your eating lifestyle is ideal. For example, heavy meat-eaters should detox every 3-4 months; Vegans would only need to detox every 6 months.

Excellent Detox Products

- Garden of Life Detox and Alkalizer
- Yogi Tea - They have a tea for skin detox as well as a general detox tea.
- Dr. Natura Detox System
- Green Tea

Excellent Detox Foods

- Broccoli
- Lemons/ Lemon water
- Neem Leaf

- Turmeric
- Garlic
- Apples
- Beetroot
- Walnuts
- Kale
- Spinach

You've seen most of these foods in other food lists. Incorporating these foods into your meals on a regular basis can help keep your intestines clean and improve fitness gains. When done properly, detoxing can be an excellent addition to your new healthy lifestyle. Just remember it is NOT a miracle cure for weight loss.

Chapter 26

Kids & Healthy Eating

Kids are the future. They are the center of our lives. We raise them and try to instill in them morals, values, and hope that our best qualities rub off on them. Unfortunately, a lot of times even our worst qualities rub off on them.

The one thing about kids that people need to understand is that they are incredibly vulnerable. They depend on their parents for everything. That's why you claim them as dependents on your taxes.

Children eat what you give them. What you eat, they eat. If you're not eating healthy, there is a good chance that your kids are not eating healthy as well. This also carries into adulthood.

Eating habits are first learned at home. When a child grows into an adult and is in a position where they have to feed themselves, they are going to do what they know. If they grew up eating a lot of fast food then there is a good chance that is how they're going to eat as an adult.

There are probably home remedies and dishes that you remember your grandmother or mother preparing that even you make to this day. That is a testament to the unique influence that parents have on their children. With this in mind, it wouldn't hurt to include your family and children in your health journey.

Chapter 27

Body Positivity: Love Yourself

In this social media-obsessed society that we live in, it's easy to get caught up in the hoopla of #BodyGoals. But the reality is that all of it is fake. Loving yourself and being as healthy as you can is the only thing that matters. When you're healthy on the inside it shows on the outside and the great thing about life is that no two people are the same. You are perfect the way you are because no one can be a better you than you.

Insecurities are normal but don't let them consume you. Only Beyonce can be Beyonce and only you can be you. Competing to be like other people is impossible and futile.

As an exercise, try this challenge: List five

things that you're grateful for in your life and list five things that you like about yourself. Every morning as you get yourself ready for the day repeat this list to yourself in the form of 'I am/ I have'. Internalize this. These are the qualities that you know that you possess. You can even add to the list if you like.

While this book was created with the intention of teaching healthy eating habits, it is important to note that self-love should be at the center of all that you do. Nothing good has ever come from chasing love or gratification outside oneself. It is impossible to please everyone. Please yourself first, and others will follow. Being happy is a choice that you must decide for yourself. Just like reading this book was a decision you made in order to lead a healthier life.

So...relax...take a breath...count down from 5... and go for it.

Live life on your terms.

Don't Forget!

Buy the Jazmin Fitness 60-day meal planner on the Jazmin Fitness website! Get organized, save money, and start eating your way to health!

JFit4Me Programs

Exercise programs for all fitness levels and guess what? It's FREE!
All programs are available on the company website.
www.JazminFitnessMembers.com

Fit4Me vMarathon

Show off your fitness journey! Sign up for our virtual marathon and send Jazmin Fitness pictures of your progress via Instagram, Twitter, or Facebook.. Win prizes, meet new people, and have fun!

About Jazmin

Jazmin Truesdale is the 'Superwoman of Superwomen'. She is the CEO, founder, and creator of the female superhero universe, Aza Comics, and is also the CEO of Jazmin Fitness. She is known to her clients as "The Fitness Doctor" and has been working as a bilingual Fitness Trainer, creating quality workout and nutrition plans in English and Spanish for over a decade.

A competitive gymnast for 9 years, she later went on to receive her degree in Exercise and Sport Science from the University of North Carolina – Chapel Hill. She is certified as a Personal Trainer through the National Academy of Sports Medicine and specializes in Women's Health and Nutrition.

Follow Jazmin for the latest fitness updates and superhero releases!

www.JazminTruesdale.com
www.AzaComics.com
Instagram: @jaztruesdale
Twitter: @JazminTruesdale

www.ingramcontent.com/pod-product-compliance
Lightning Source LLC
Chambersburg PA
CBHW021100210326
41598CB00016B/1272